OSTEOPOROSIS

Juicing & Smoothies

For Seniors

BONUS

10 Herbs For Bone

Health Plus

Meal

Planner

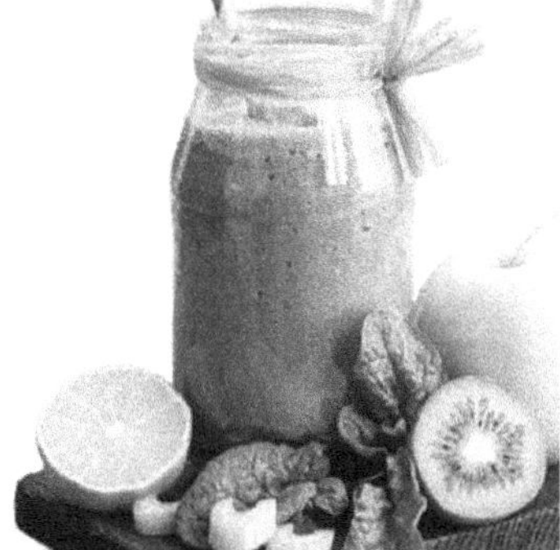

The Ultimate Nutrient Dense Recipes For Stronger Bones, Easy Absorption, And Optimal Health

LEONA BUTLER

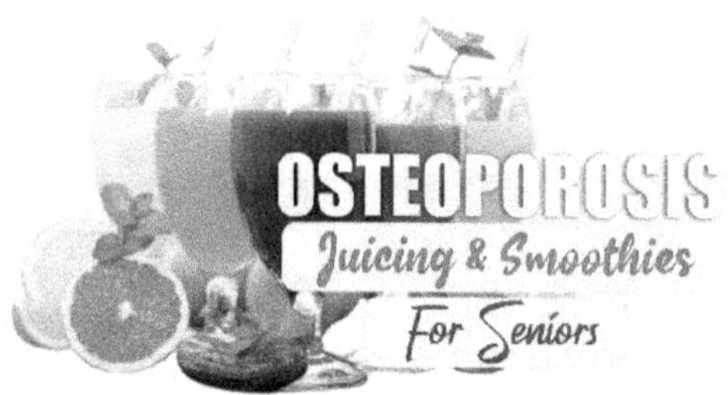
OSTEOPOROSIS
Juicing & Smoothies
For Seniors

1. Understand Nutrient Needs: Research and understand the nutrients beneficial for bone health, such as calcium, vitamin D, vitamin K, magnesium, and phosphorus.

2. Select Ingredients: Choose ingredients rich in these nutrients. For example, leafy greens like kale and spinach are high in calcium and vitamin K, while dairy or fortified non-dairy milk can provide calcium and vitamin D. Fruits like oranges and berries can add flavor and additional nutrients.

3. Plan Recipes: Look for smoothie and juicing recipes specifically designed for osteoporosis. These recipes often incorporate ingredients known for their bone-strengthening properties.

4. Prepare Ingredients: Wash and prepare all fruits and vegetables. If using fresh fruits, remove any seeds or pits. If using frozen ingredients, allow them to thaw slightly for easier blending.

5. Blend or Juice: Follow the recipe instructions to blend or juice the ingredients together until smooth. If necessary, add liquid (such as water, milk, or juice) to achieve the desired consistency.

6. Enjoy Regularly: Incorporate these smoothies or juices into your daily routine. Aim to consume them consistently to provide your body with a steady supply of bone-boosting nutrients.

7. Monitor and Adjust: Pay attention to how your body responds to these recipes. If you notice improvements in your bone health or overall well-being, continue enjoying them. If you have any concerns or encounter any side effects, speak with a healthcare practitioner for personalized advice. By following these steps, you can effectively use smoothie and juicing recipes to support your bone health and manage osteoporosis.

TABLE OF CONTENT

3. 10 MAGNESIUM AND PHOSPHORUS-PACKED SMOOTHIES:

1. BANANA AND ALMOND BUTTER SMOOTHIE:
2. QUINOA AND BERRY SMOOTHIE:
3. PUMPKIN SEED AND SPINACH SHAKE:
4. OATMEAL AND FIG SMOOTHIE:
5. BLACK BEAN AND COCOA SMOOTHIE:
6. CASHEW AND DATE SHAKE:
7. BROWN RICE AND BANANA SMOOTHIE:
8. LENTIL AND MANGO SHAKE:
9. SESAME SEED AND APRICOT SMOOTHIE:
10. CHIA SEED AND PRUNE SHAKE:

4. BONUS: HERBAL AND SUPPLEMENTAL ADDITIONS

HERBS FOR BONE HEALTH

1. TURMERIC:
2. GINGER:
3. NETTLE:
4. HORSETAIL:
5. DANDELION:
6. OREGANO:
7. BASIL:

5. BONUS 2: WEEKS MEAL PLANNER

THE PAPERBACK OF THIS VERSION HAS A WEEKS MEAL PLANNER

CONCLUSION

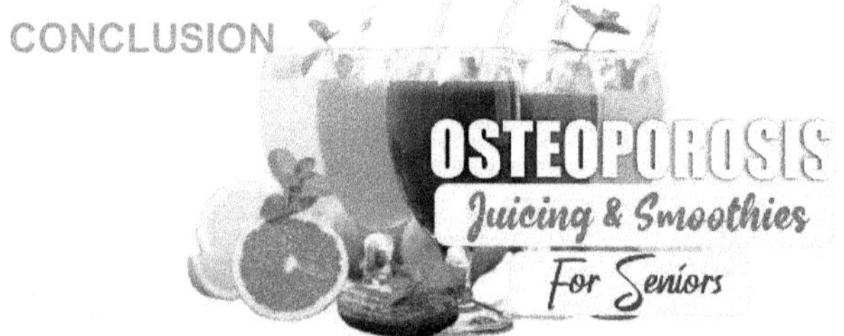

Introduction

Unlocking Bone Health: Harnessing the Power of Smoothies and Juicing for Osteoporosis" introduces a comprehensive approach to combating osteoporosis through the delicious and nutritious world of smoothies and juices.

In this book, readers will discover the myriad benefits these vibrant beverages offer, tailored specifically to support bone health. By delving into the nutrient density of carefully selected ingredients like leafy greens, fruits, nuts, and seeds, individuals can tap into a treasure trove of essential vitamins and minerals crucial for fortifying bones against osteoporosis.

The easy absorption of nutrients provided by blending or juicing ensures that even those with compromised digestive systems can reap the rewards. Moreover, the alkalizing properties of these concoctions help counteract acidity in the body, potentially reducing calcium loss from bones.

As hydration is paramount for bone strength, the book emphasizes the importance of incorporating smoothies and juices into daily routines. Additionally, by promoting weight management, antioxidant protection, and fiber intake, these beverages offer a holistic approach to bone health that is both convenient and delicious. "Unlocking Bone Health" is not just a recipe book—it's a guide to transforming lifestyles and fostering lasting vitality through the simple joy of sipping on nature's bounty.

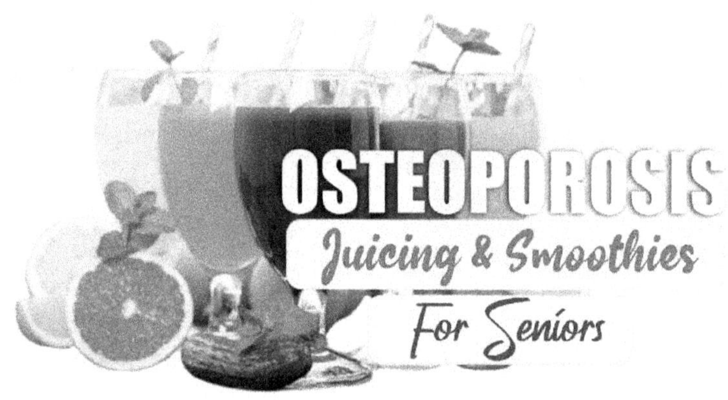

1. Basics of Juicing and Smoothies

Juicing and smoothies are popular methods of consuming fruits and vegetables in a convenient and tasty way. Juicing involves extracting the liquid from fruits and vegetables, leaving behind the pulp, while smoothies blend the whole fruits and vegetables, including the fiber. Both methods offer a convenient means to increase nutrient intake and promote overall health.

Benefits of Juicing and Smoothies

1. Nutrient Absorption: Juicing and smoothies allow for easy absorption of nutrients since the fruits and vegetables are broken down into a liquid form, making it easier for the body to digest and absorb essential vitamins and minerals.

2. Increased Fruit and Vegetable Consumption: Many people struggle to meet their recommended daily intake of fruits and vegetables. Juicing and smoothies provide a convenient way to increase consumption, helping individuals meet their nutritional needs.

3. Hydration: Both juicing and smoothies contribute to hydration since they primarily consist of water-rich fruits and vegetables. Staying hydrated is crucial for overall health and well-being.

4. Digestive Health: The fiber content in smoothies aids in digestion and promotes a healthy gut microbiome. Juicing, while lower in fiber, can still provide some digestive benefits, particularly for individuals with digestive issues.

5. Boosted Immunity: Fruits and vegetables are rich in vitamins, minerals, and antioxidants, which support the immune system and help the body fight off infections and diseases.

6. Weight Management: Juicing and smoothies can be incorporated into a balanced diet to support weight management efforts. They provide a low-calorie option for satisfying cravings and can help prevent overeating.

When preparing juices and smoothies, it's essential to select fresh, high-quality ingredients to maximize nutritional benefits. Opt for a variety of fruits and vegetables to ensure a diverse nutrient profile. Incorporating leafy greens, such as spinach or kale, adds vitamins and minerals without significantly impacting the flavor. Additionally, including a source of protein, such as Greek yogurt or plant-based protein powder, can help balance blood sugar levels and promote satiety. Be mindful of added sugars, opting for natural sweeteners like honey or dates if sweetness is desired.

Equipment and Preparation Tips

Investing in a high-quality juicer or blender is key to achieving smooth and consistent results. Centrifugal juicers are ideal for beginners and are suitable for most fruits and vegetables, while masticating juicers are better for leafy greens and produce higher juice yields. For smoothies, a powerful blender capable of crushing ice and frozen ingredients is essential. To save time, prep ingredients in advance by washing, peeling, and chopping fruits and vegetables, then storing them in portioned bags or containers in the fridge or freezer. Experiment with different combinations of ingredients to find flavors and textures that appeal to your preferences.

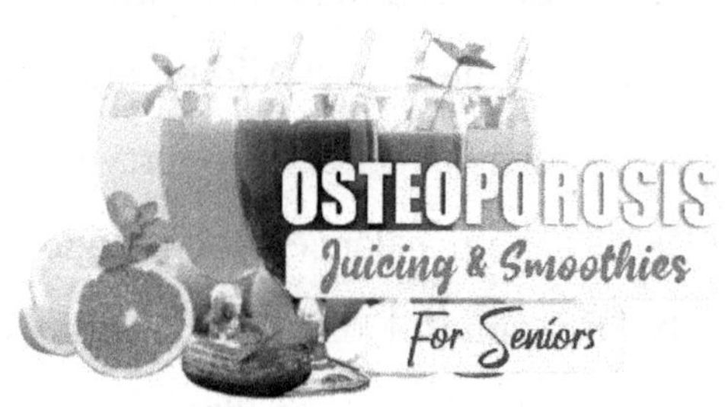

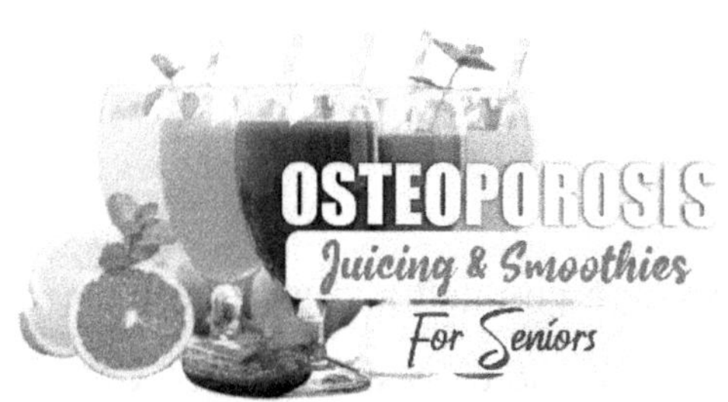

1. 10 Recipes for Calcium-Rich Drinks:

1. Orange Creamsicle Smoothie

Ingredients:

- 1 cup fresh orange juice
- 1/2 cup Greek yogurt
- 1/2 cup unsweetened almond milk
- 1 ripe banana
- 1/2 teaspoon vanilla extract
- 1 tablespoon honey or maple syrup (optional)
- Ice cubes (optional)

Preparation:

1. Peel and chop the banana.
2. Combine all the ingredients in a blender.
3. Blend until smooth and creamy.
4. Add ice cubes if desired for a colder texture.

Nutritional Value:

- Calories: Approximately 220
- Protein: 8g
- Fat: 2g
- Carbohydrates: 45g
- Fiber: 4g
- Vitamin C: 150% DV

2. Almond Milk and Date Shake

Ingredients:

- 1 cup unsweetened almond milk
- 4-5 pitted dates
- 1/4 teaspoon cinnamon
- 1/2 teaspoon vanilla extract
- Ice cubes

Preparation:

1. Soak the pitted dates in warm water for about 10 minutes
   to soften them.

2. Drain the dates and place them in a blender.

3. Add almond milk, cinnamon, and vanilla extract.

4. Blend until smooth.

5. Add ice cubes and blend again for a colder shake.

Nutritional Value:

- Calories: Approximately 160

- Protein: 1g

- Fat: 3g

- Carbohydrates: 35g

- Fiber: 4g

3. Tropical Green Smoothie

Ingredients:

- 1 cup coconut water

- 1 cup spinach leaves

- 1/2 cup frozen pineapple chunks

- 1/2 cup frozen mango chunks

- 1/2 banana

- Juice of 1/2 lime

- Optional: 1 tablespoon chia seeds

Preparation:

1. Place all the ingredients in a blender.
2. Blend until smooth.
3. Add more coconut water as needed to achieve the desired consistency.

Nutritional Value:

- Calories: Approximately 180
- Protein: 4g
- Fat: 1g
- Carbohydrates: 45g
- Fiber: 8g
- Vitamin C: 200% DV

Ingredients:

- 1 cup frozen strawberries
- 1/2 cup Greek yogurt
- 1/2 cup unsweetened almond milk
- 1 tablespoon honey or maple syrup (optional) Ice cubes (optional)

Preparation:

1. Combine all the ingredients in a blender.
2. Blend until smooth.
3. Add ice cubes if desired for a colder texture.

Nutritional Value:

- Calories: Approximately 160
- Protein: 8g
- Fat: 2g
- Carbohydrates: 30g

- Fiber: 5g
- Vitamin C: 150% DV

Enjoy your nutritious and delicious smoothies!

5. Berry Blast Calcium Smoothie:

Ingredients:

- cup of mixed berries (strawberries, blueberries, raspberries) cup of spinach
- 1/2 cup of plain Greek yogurt
- 1 tablespoon of honey
- 1 cup of almond milk 1 tablespoon of chia seeds

Method:

1. Combine all ingredients in a blender.
2. Blend until smooth and creamy.
3. Serve immediately.

Nutritional Value: High in antioxidants, vitamins, and minerals. Provides a good dose of calcium from the yogurt and almond milk.

Ingredients:

- 2 ripe bananas
- 2 cups of chopped collard greens
- 1/2 cup of almond milk
- 1 tablespoon of almond butter 1 tablespoon of honey

Method:

- Place all ingredients in a blender.
- Blend until smooth.
- Serve chilled.

Nutritional Value: Rich in potassium, fiber, and vitamins A and C. Provides a good source of calcium and healthy fats from almond milk and almond butter.

7. Chia Seed Pudding:

Ingredients:

- 1/4 cup of chia seeds
- 1 cup almond milk (or other milk of your choosing)
- 1 tablespoon of honey or maple syrup 1/2 teaspoon of vanilla extract

Method:

1. In a bowl, mix chia seeds, almond milk, honey, and vanilla extract.
2. Stir well to combine.
3. Cover and refrigerate for at least 2 hours or overnight, until thickened.
4. Serve chilled, topped with fruits or nuts if desired.

Nutritional Value: High in fiber, omega-3 fatty acids, and protein. Provides a good source of calcium and antioxidants.

Ingredients:

- ripe avocado ripe banana
- 2 tablespoons of cocoa powder
- 1 cup of almond milk
- 1 tablespoon of honey or maple syrup (optional, adjust to taste)

Method:

1. Scoop the flesh of the avocado and banana into a blender.
2. Add cocoa powder, almond milk, and sweetener if using.
3. Blend until smooth and creamy.
4. Serve immediately.

Nutritional Value: Rich in healthy fats, potassium, and antioxidants. Provides a good source of calcium and magnesium from almond milk and cocoa powder.

9. Peaches and Cream Smoothie:

Ingredients:

- 1 cup frozen peaches
- 1/2 cup Greek yogurt
- 1/2 cup almond milk
- 1 tablespoon honey
- 1/2 teaspoon vanilla extract Ice cubes (optional)

Preparation:

1. Place frozen peaches, Greek yogurt, almond milk, honey, and vanilla extract in a blender.
2. Blend until smooth.
3. If desired, add ice cubes and blend again until desired consistency is reached.
4. Serve immediately.

Nutritional Value (per serving):
- Calories: 180
- Protein: 10g

- Carbohydrates: 30g

- Fat: 3g

- Fiber: 3g

10. Cottage Cheese and Spinach Shake:

Ingredients:

- 1/2 cup cottage cheese

- 1 cup fresh spinach leaves

- 1/2 banana

- 1/2 cup unsweetened almond milk

- tablespoon chia seeds

- teaspoon honey or maple syrup (optional) Ice cubes (optional)

Preparation:

1. Combine cottage cheese, spinach leaves, banana, almond milk, chia seeds, and honey/maple syrup (if using) in a blender.
2. Blend until smooth.

3. If desired, add ice cubes and blend again until desired consistency is reached. Serve immediately.

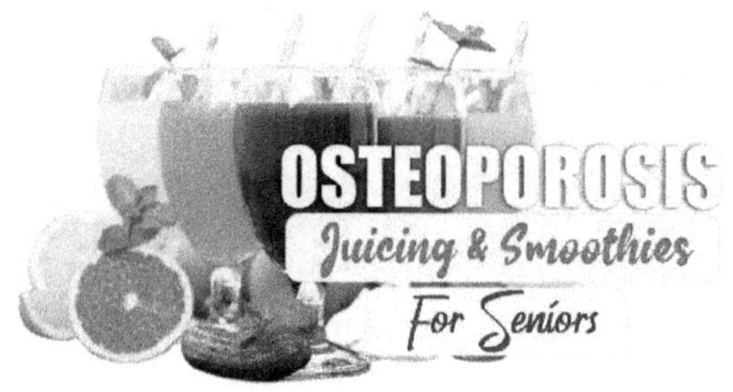

2. 10 Vitamin D Boosting Blends

1. Sunshine Smoothie:

Ingredients:

- 1 cup of fresh orange juice
- 1 banana, sliced
- 1/2 cup of pineapple chunks
- 1/2 cup of Greek yogurt
- 1 tablespoon of honey Ice cubes (optional)

Preparation:

1. In a blender, combine the fresh orange juice, sliced banana, pineapple chunks, Greek yogurt, and honey.
2. Blend until smooth and creamy.
3. If desired, add ice cubes and mix again until well combined.
4. Serve immediately and enjoy! Nutritional Value:
5. Provides vitamin C from oranges and pineapple.
6. Potassium from banana.
7. Protein from Greek yogurt. Natural sugars for energy.

2. Salmon and Avocado Smoothie:

Ingredients:

- 4 oz cooked salmon fillet, chilled
- 1/2 ripe avocado, peeled and pitted
- 1 cup of spinach leaves
- 1/2 cup of cucumber, diced
- 1/4 cup of plain yogurt
- 1/2 cup of almond milk Salt and pepper to taste

Preparation:

1. In a blender, combine the cooked salmon, avocado, spinach leaves, diced cucumber, plain yogurt, and almond milk.
2. Season with salt and pepper to taste.
3. Blend until smooth and creamy.
4. Pour into a glass and serve chilled.

Nutritional Value:

- Provides omega-3 fatty acids from salmon.
- Healthy fats from avocado.
- Vitamins and minerals from spinach and cucumber. Protein from yogurt.

3. Mushroom and Kale Shake

Ingredients:

- 1 cup of kale leaves, stems removed
- 1/2 cup of cooked mushrooms
- 1/2 ripe banana
- 1 tablespoon of almond butter
- 1 cup of unsweetened almond milk Dash of cinnamon (optional)

Preparation:

1. In a blender, combine the kale leaves, cooked mushrooms, ripe banana, almond butter, and unsweetened almond milk.

2. Add a dash of cinnamon if desired.

3. Blend until smooth and creamy.

4. Pour into a glass and serve immediately. Nutritional Value:

5. Provides antioxidants and vitamins from kale and mushrooms.

6. Potassium and fiber from banana.

7. Healthy fats from almond butter. Low in sugar.

4. Fortified Cereal Smoothie:

Ingredients:

- 1 cup of fortified cereal (such as bran flakes or whole grain cereal)
- 1 cup of unsweetened almond milk
- 1/2 cup of frozen mixed berries
- 1/2 banana
- 1 tablespoon of chia seeds

Preparation:

1. In a blender, combine the fortified cereal, unsweetened almond milk, frozen mixed berries, banana, and chia seeds.
2. Blend until smooth and well combined.
3. If too thick, add more almond milk as needed.
4. Pour into a glass and serve immediately.

Nutritional Value:

- Provides fiber, vitamins, and minerals from fortified cereal.
- Antioxidants and vitamins from mixed berries.
- Potassium and fiber from banana.
- Chia seeds include both omega-3 fatty acids and fiber.

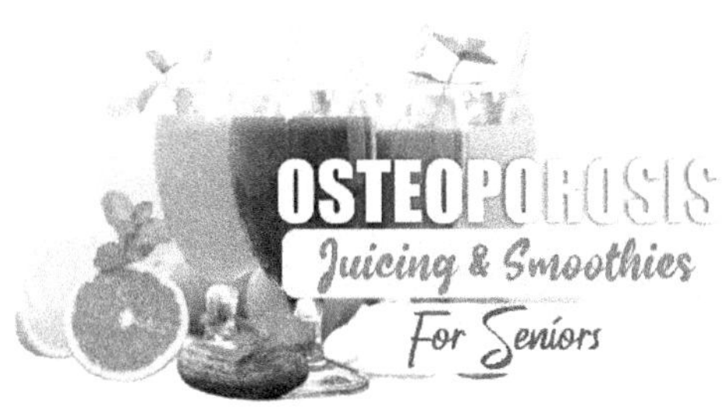

5. Egg Yolk and Spinach Smoothie:

Ingredients:

- 1 cup fresh spinach leaves
- 1 ripe banana
- 1 egg yolk
- 1/2 cup Greek yogurt
- 1/2 cup almond milk
- 1 tablespoon honey Ice cubes (optional)

Preparation:

1. Wash the spinach leaves thoroughly.
2. Peel and slice the ripe banana.
3. In a blender, combine the spinach leaves, sliced banana, egg yolk, Greek yogurt, almond milk, and honey.
4. Blend until smooth and creamy.
5. If required, add more ice cubes and mix until smooth.
6. Pour into glasses and serve immediately.

Nutritional Value:

- Calories: Approx. 250
- Protein: Approx. 10g
- Fiber: Approx. 5g
- Vitamins and Minerals: High in Vitamin A, Vitamin C, Calcium, and Iron

6. Tuna and Spinach Shake:

Ingredients:

- 1 cup fresh spinach leaves
- 1 small can of tuna in water (about 3-4 ounces)
- 1/2 avocado
- 1/2 cup unsweetened almond milk
- 1 tablespoon lemon juice
- Salt and pepper to taste Ice cubes (optional)

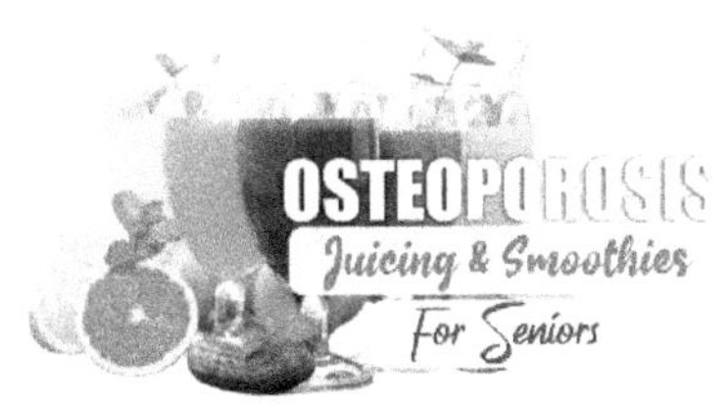

Preparation:

1. Wash the spinach leaves thoroughly. Drain the water from the can of tuna.
2. In a blender, combine the spinach leaves, drained tuna, avocado, almond milk, lemon juice, salt, and pepper.
3. Blend until smooth and well combined.
4. If required, add more ice cubes and mix until smooth.
5. Pour into glasses and serve chilled.

Nutritional Value:

- Calories: Approx. 300
- Protein: Approx. 25g
- Fiber: Approx. 7g
- Healthy Fats: Avocado provides healthy monounsaturated fats
- Omega-3 Fatty Acids: Tuna is rich in omega-3 fatty acids, which are beneficial for heart health.

Ingredients:

- 1 cup shiitake mushrooms, sliced
- 1 cup vegetable broth
- 1/2 cup unsweetened almond milk
- 1/4 cup plain Greek yogurt
- 1/2 teaspoon minced garlic 1/2 teaspoon grated ginger
- 1 tablespoon nutritional yeast Salt and pepper to taste

Preparation:

1. In a saucepan, combine the sliced shiitake mushrooms, vegetable broth, minced garlic, and grated ginger.
2. Bring the mixture to a simmer over medium heat and cook for about 10 minutes, or until the mushrooms are tender.
3. Remove the saucepan from the heat and let the mixture cool slightly.
4. Transfer the mushroom mixture to a blender and add the unsweetened almond milk, plain Greek yogurt, nutritional yeast, salt, and pepper.

5. Blend until smooth and creamy.

6. Serve warm or chilled, depending on preference.

Nutritional Value:

- This smoothie is rich in protein from the Greek yogurt and almond milk.

- Shiitake mushrooms provide essential vitamins and minerals like vitamin D, B vitamins, and selenium.

- Nutritional yeast adds a cheesy flavor and is a source of B vitamins, particularly vitamin B12 for vegans or vegetarians.

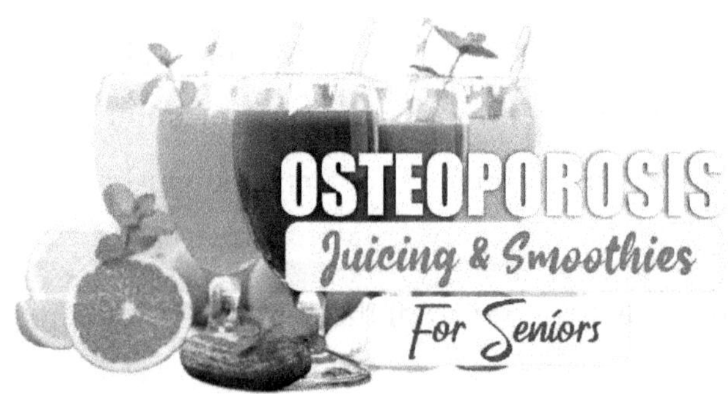

Ingredients:

- 1 cup spinach
- 1/2 cup frozen berries (such as strawberries, blueberries, or raspberries)
- 1/2 banana
- 1 tablespoon cod liver oil
- 1/2 cup unsweetened coconut water
- 1/4 cup plain Greek yogurt

Preparation:

1. Place all ingredients in a blender.
2. Blend until smooth and creamy.
3. Adjust the consistency by adding more coconut water if necessary.
4. Serve immediately.

Nutritional Value:

1. This smoothie is packed with antioxidants from the spinach and berries.
2. Cod liver oil is rich in omega-3 fatty acids, vitamins A and D, which are essential for overall health, particularly for brain function, vision, and immune system support. Greek yogurt adds protein and probiotics, beneficial for gut health.

9. Sardine and Kale Smoothie:

Ingredients:

- 1 cup kale leaves, washed and chopped
- 1 small ripe banana, peeled and sliced
- 1/2 cup frozen pineapple chunks
- 1/4 cup plain Greek yogurt
- 1/4 cup almond milk
- 1 tablespoon chia seeds
- 1 can (3.75 oz) sardines in water, drained
- 1 teaspoon honey (optional) Ice cubes (optional)

Preparation:

1. In a blender, combine the kale, banana, pineapple chunks, Greek yogurt, almond milk, chia seeds, and drained sardines.
2. Blend on high speed until smooth and creamy, adding honey if desired for sweetness.
3. If a thicker consistency is preferred, add ice cubes and blend again until smooth.
4. Pour into a glass and enjoy immediately.

Nutritional Value:

- Calories: Approximately 320
- Protein: Approximately 24 grams
- Fat: Approximately 14 grams
- Carbohydrates: Approximately 26 grams
- Fiber: Approximately 7 grams

10. Swiss Cheese and Spinach Shake:

Ingredients:

- 1 cup fresh spinach leaves, washed
- 1/2 cup sliced cucumber
- 1/2 cup sliced avocado
- 1/4 cup shredded Swiss cheese
- 1/4 cup plain Greek yogurt
- 1/2 cup almond milk
- 1 tablespoon lemon juice
- 1/4 teaspoon ground black pepper Ice cubes (optional)

Preparation:

1. In a blender, combine the spinach leaves, sliced cucumber, avocado, shredded Swiss cheese, Greek yogurt, almond milk, lemon juice, and ground black pepper. Blend at high speeds until smooth and creamy.
2. If a colder temperature is desired, add ice cubes and blend again until smooth.
3. Pour into a glass and serve immediately.

3. 10 Magnesium and Phosphorus-Packed Smoothies:

1. Banana and Almond Butter Smoothie:

Ingredients:

- ripe banana
- tablespoons almond butter
- 1 cup almond milk
- 1/2 cup Greek yogurt
- 1 tablespoon honey (optional) Ice cubes (optional)

Preparation:

1. Peel the banana and cut into bits.
2. In a blender, combine the banana chunks, almond butter, almond milk, Greek yogurt, and honey
3. (if using).
4. Blend until smooth and creamy.
5. If required, add more ice cubes and mix until smooth.
6. Pour into glasses and serve immediately.

Nutritional Value (per serving):

- Calories: 280

- Protein: 11g

- Fat: 14g

- Carbohydrates: 30g

- Fiber: 5g

- Sugar: 17g

2. Quinoa and Berry Smoothie:

Ingredients:

- 1/2 cup cooked quinoa

- 1 cup mixed berries (such as strawberries, blueberries, raspberries)

- 1/2 cup spinach leaves

- 1 cup almond milk

- 1 tablespoon honey (optional) Ice cubes (optional)

Preparation:

1. Cook the quinoa according to the package directions and let it cool.
2. In a blender, combine the cooked quinoa, mixed berries, spinach leaves, almond milk, and honey (if using).
3. Blend until smooth.
4. If preferred, add ice cubes and mix until smooth.
5. Pour into glasses and serve immediately.

Nutritional Value (per serving):

- Calories: 230
- Protein: 8g
- Fat: 4g
- Carbohydrates: 45g
- Fiber: 7g
- Sugar: 15g

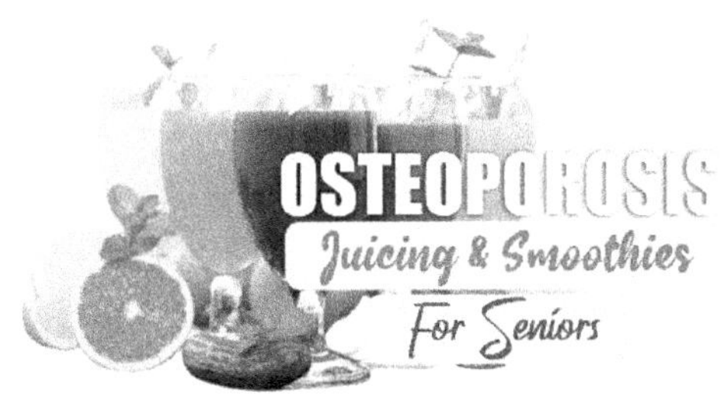

3. Pumpkin Seed and Spinach Shake:

Ingredients:

- 1/4 cup pumpkin seeds
- 1 cup spinach leaves
- 1 ripe banana
- 1 cup almond milk
- 1 tablespoon honey (optional) Ice cubes (optional)

Preparation:

1. In a blender, combine the pumpkin seeds, spinach leaves, banana, almond milk, and honey (if using).
2. Blend until smooth.
3. If required, add more ice cubes and mix until smooth.
4. Pour into glasses and serve immediately.

Nutritional Value (per serving):

- Calories: 220
- Protein: 9g
- Fat: 10g
- Carbohydrates: 28g

- Fiber: 5g
- Sugar: 15g

Enjoy your nutritious smoothies!

4. Oatmeal and Fig Smoothie:

Ingredients:

- 1/2 cup rolled oats
- 2 dried figs, stems removed
- 1 ripe banana
- 1 cup almond milk
- 1 tablespoon honey or maple syrup (optional) Ice cubes (optional)

Preparation:

1. In a blender, combine rolled oats, dried figs, ripe banana, almond milk, and honey or maple syrup if using.
2. Blend until smooth and creamy.
3. If you want your smoothie colder, add some ice cubes.
4. Pour into glasses and serve immediately.

Nutritional Value:

This smoothie is rich in fiber from oats and figs, potassium from banana, and healthy fats from almond milk, making it a nutritious and filling breakfast option.

5. Black Bean and Cocoa Smoothie:

Ingredients:

- 1/2 cup cooked black beans
- 1 tablespoon cocoa powder
- 1 ripe banana
- 1 cup milk (dairy or plant-based)
- 1 tablespoon honey or maple syrup (optional) Ice cubes (optional)

Preparation:

1. Combine cooked black beans, cocoa powder, ripe banana, milk, and honey or maple syrup if using, in a blender.
2. Blend until smooth and well combined.

3. Add ice cubes if desired for a thicker texture and colder temperature.
4. Pour into glasses and serve immediately.

Nutritional Value:

This smoothie is packed with protein from black beans, antioxidants from cocoa powder, potassium from banana, and calcium from milk, making it a nutritious post-workout or snack option.

6. Cashew and Date Shake:

Ingredients:
- 1/4 cup cashews, soaked overnight
- 2-3 dates, pitted
- 1 ripe banana
- 1 cup coconut milk
- 1/2 teaspoon vanilla extract Ice cubes (optional)

Preparation:

- Drain and rinse soaked cashews.

- In a blender, combine soaked cashews, pitted dates, ripe banana, coconut milk, and vanilla extract.

- Blend until smooth and creamy.

- Add ice cubes if desired for a colder shake.

- Pour into glasses and serve immediately.

Nutritional Value:

This shake is rich in healthy fats and protein from cashews, natural sweetness from dates, potassium from banana, and medium-chain triglycerides from coconut milk, making it a satisfying and nourishing beverage.

7. Brown Rice and Banana Smoothie:

Ingredients:

- 1/2 cup cooked brown rice

- 1 ripe banana

- 1 cup almond milk (or any milk you want)

- 1 tablespoon honey (optional) 1/2 teaspoon vanilla extract (optional)

Preparation:

1. In a blender, combine the cooked brown rice, ripe banana, almond milk, honey, and vanilla extract.
2. Blend until smooth and creamy.
3. Pour into glasses and serve immediately.

Nutritional Value:

- Brown rice: High in fiber, vitamins, and minerals such as manganese and magnesium.
- Banana is high in potassium, vitamin C, and vitamin B6.
- Almond milk is rich in vitamin E and calcium.
- Honey contains antioxidants and may possess antimicrobial qualities. Vanilla extract: Provides flavor without adding calories or fat.

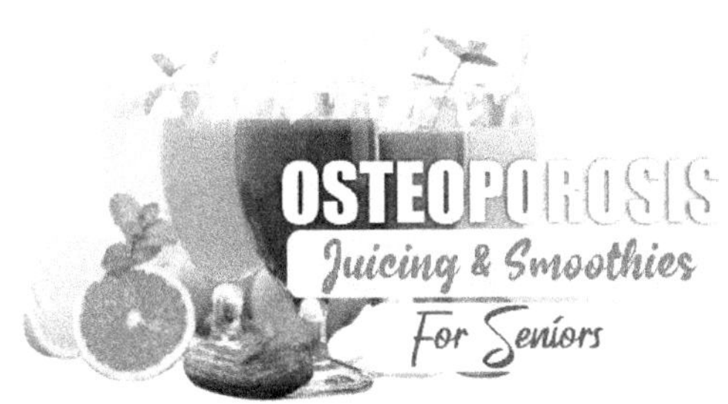

8. Lentil and Mango Shake:

Ingredients:

- 1/2 cup cooked lentils (any variety)
- 1 ripe mango, peeled and diced
- 1 cup coconut water (or regular water)
- 1 tablespoon lime juice
- 1 tablespoon maple syrup or agave syrup (optional)

Preparation:

1. In a blender, combine the cooked lentils, diced mango, coconut water, lime juice, and maple syrup.
2. Blend until smooth and well combined.
3. Taste and adjust the sweetness as needed by adding more maple syrup.
4. Pour into glasses and serve chilled.

9. Sesame Seed and Apricot Smoothie:

Ingredients:

- 2 tablespoons sesame seeds
- 1 cup ripe apricots, pitted
- 1/2 cup Greek yogurt (or dairy-free yogurt for vegan option) 1 cup unsweetened almond milk (or any milk you want)
- 1 tablespoon honey or maple syrup (optional)

Preparation:

1. In a blender, combine the sesame seeds, ripe apricots, Greek yogurt, almond milk, and honey or maple syrup.
2. Blend until smooth and creamy.
3. Taste and adjust the sweetness as needed by adding more honey or maple syrup.
4. Pour into glasses and serve chilled.

10. Chia Seed and Prune Shake:

Ingredients:

- 2 tablespoons of chia seeds
- 4-5 prunes, pitted
- 1 cup almond milk (or other milk of your choosing)
- 1 teaspoon of honey (optional, for sweetness) Ice cubes (optional, for a chilled shake)

Preparation:

1. Soak the chia seeds in 1/4 cup of water for about 10-15 minutes until they form a gel-like consistency.
2. In a blender, combine the soaked chia seeds, pitted prunes, almond milk, and honey.
3. Blend until smooth and creamy. If preferred, add ice and blend until smooth. Pour the mix into glasses and serve instantly.

4. BONUS: Herbal and Supplemental Additions

Herbs for Bone Health

1. Turmeric:

Ingredients:

- 1 tablespoon of ground turmeric
- 1 cup of water or milk
- Honey or sweetener to taste (optional)

Preparation:

1. Heat the water or milk in a saucepan until it starts to simmer.
2. Add the ground turmeric and stir well.
3. Allow it to simmer for around 10 minutes, stirring occasionally. Strain the mixture to exclude any solid particles.
4. Sweeten with honey if desired.

2. Ginger:

Ingredients:

- 1 tablespoon of grated fresh ginger
- 1 cup of water
- Honey or sweetener to taste (optional)

Preparation:

1. Boil the water in a saucepan.
2. Add the grated ginger to the boiling water. Let it simmer for 5-10 minutes.
3. Strain the mixture to remove the ginger.
4. Sweeten with honey if desired.

Nutritional Value:

- Ginger includes gingerol, a bioactive molecule that has strong anti-inflammatory and antioxidant properties.
- It also provides essential nutrients like vitamin C, potassium, and magnesium.

Ingredients:

- 1 tablespoon of dried nettle leaves 1 cup of boiling water
- Lemon or honey to taste (optional)

Preparation:

1. Place the dried nettle leaves in a cup.
2. Pour the boiling water on the nettle leaves.
3. Let it steep for 5-10 minutes.
4. Strain the mixture to remove the leaves.
5. Add lemon or honey if desired.

Nutritional Value:

Nettle is rich in vitamins A, C, and K, as well as minerals like iron and calcium. It also has antioxidant properties and may help reduce inflammation.

4. Horsetail:

Ingredients:

- 1 tablespoon of dried horsetail herb
- 1 cup of hot water
- Lemon or honey to taste (optional)

Preparation:

1. Place the dried horsetail herb in a cup.
2. Pour the hot water over the herb.
3. Let it steep for 10-15 minutes.
4. Strain the mixture to remove the herb.
5. Add lemon or honey if desired.

Nutritional Value:

- Horsetail is rich in silica, which may promote hair, skin, and nail health.
- It contains antioxidants and has diuretic qualities. However, it should be consumed in moderation due to its potential for toxicity in large amounts.

5. Dandelion:

Ingredients:

- Wash and cut two cups of fresh dandelion greens.
- tablespoon olive oil
- cloves garlic, minced Salt and pepper to taste

Preparation:

1. In a medium-sized pan, heat the olive oil.
2. Add minced garlic and sauté until fragrant.
3. Add chopped dandelion greens and cook for 3-5 minutes until wilted.
4. Season with salt and pepper to taste.
5. Serve hot.

Nutritional Value:

Dandelion greens are low in calories and high in fiber, vitamins A, C, and K, as well as several minerals including calcium, iron, and potassium.

6. Oregano:

Ingredients:

- 2 tablespoons dried oregano leaves
- 1 tablespoon olive oil
- Salt to taste

Preparation:

1. Preheat oven to 250°F (120°C).
2. In a bowl, mix dried oregano leaves with olive oil until well coated.
3. Spread the oregano mixture on a baking sheet lined with parchment paper.
4. Bake for 10-15 minutes until the leaves are crispy.
5. Remove from the oven, sprinkle with salt, and let cool.
6. Store in an airtight container.

Nutritional Value:

Oregano contains antioxidants, vitamins A, C, and K, and minerals such as calcium, iron, and manganese.

Ingredients:

- cup fresh basil leaves
- tablespoons pine nuts
- 2 cloves garlic
- ¼ cup grated Parmesan cheese
- ¼ cup olive oil
- Salt and pepper to taste

Preparation:

1. In a food processor, combine the basil leaves, pine nuts, garlic, and Parmesan cheese. Pulse until finely chopped.
2. While the machine is running, gently add olive oil until the mixture reaches a smooth consistency.
3. Season with salt and pepper to taste.
4. Serve with pasta, as a spread, or use as a topping for various dishes.

Nutritional Value:

Basil is rich in vitamins A, K, and C, as well as magnesium, iron, potassium, and calcium.

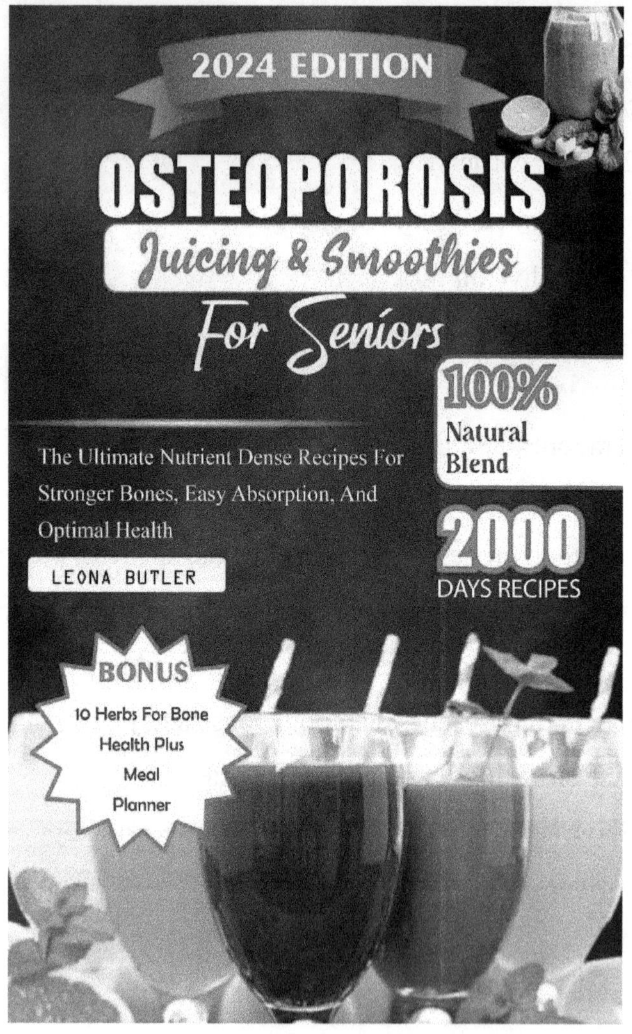

BONUS 2: weeks meal planner

The Paperback of This Version Has a Weeks Meal Planner

MY WEEKLY MEAL PLANNER

Date

	Breakfast	Lunch	Dinner
MON			
TUE			
WED			
THU			
FRI			
SAT			
SUN			

SHOPPING LIST:

To Do List

NOTES AND TIPS

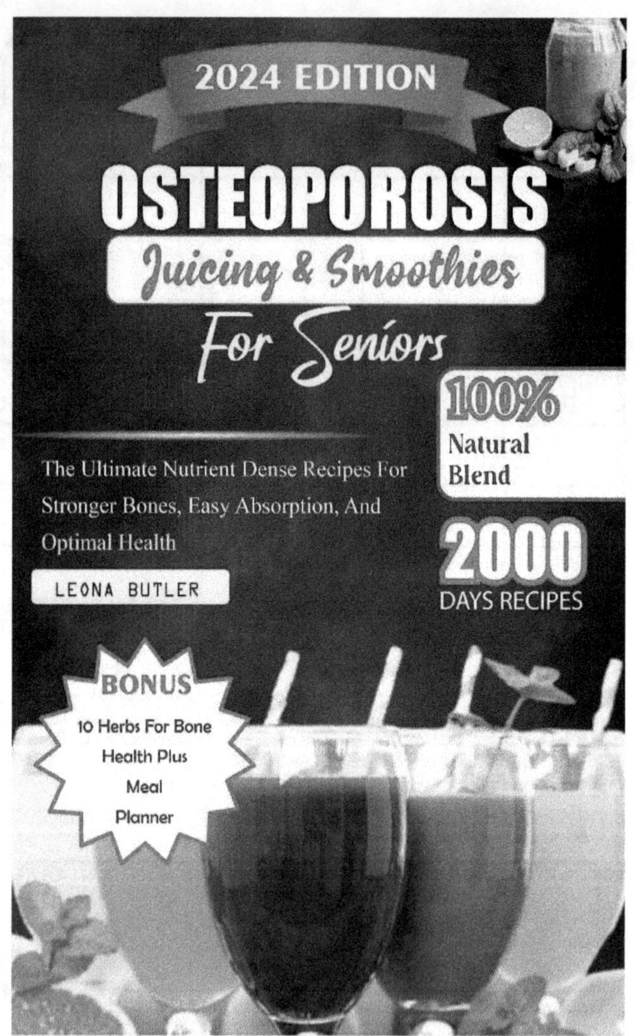

2024 EDITION
OSTEOPOROSIS
Juicing & Smoothies
For Seniors
100%
Natural
Blend
The Ultimate Nutrient Dense Recipes For
Stronger Bones, Easy Absorption, And
Optimal Health
LEONA BUTLER
2000
DAYS RECIPES
BONUS
10 Herbs For Bone
Health Plus
Meal
Planner

Conclusion

Smoothies and Juicing for Osteoporosis" offers a holistic approach to bone health through the power of nutrient-rich beverages. By harnessing the benefits of smoothies and juices, individuals can nourish their bodies with essential vitamins and minerals crucial for bone strength.

These beverages provide a convenient and enjoyable way to incorporate a variety of bone-healthy ingredients into the diet, supporting optimal nutrition for those managing osteoporosis.

From calcium-rich leafy greens to vitamin D-packed fruits, each sip delivers hydration, alkalizing properties, and easy-to-absorb nutrients, vital for maintaining bone density. Moreover, the antioxidant protection and fiber content found in these beverages contribute to overall health, reducing inflammation, supporting digestion, and promoting weight management—key factors in preventing fractures and enhancing bone resilience.

Smoothies and Juicing for Osteoporosis" empowers readers to take control of their bone health with delicious and nutritious recipes, offering a flavorful path to stronger bones and a vibrant life.

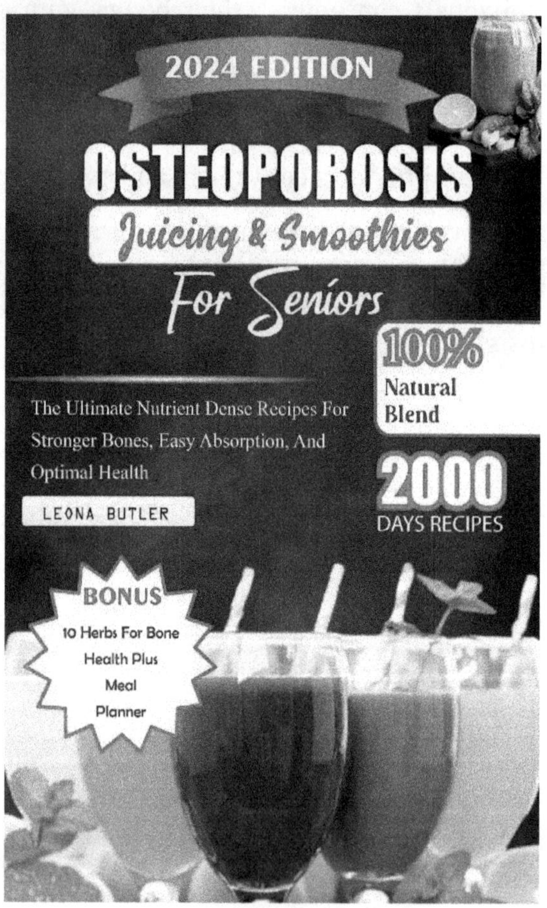

Thank you

Thank you for embarking on this journey towards better bone health with "Smoothies and Juicing for Osteoporosis." Your commitment to exploring holistic approaches to wellness is commendable, and I hope this book has provided you with valuable insights and practical strategies for nourishing your body from within.

By delving into the world of nutrient-rich beverages, you've taken a proactive step towards supporting your bones and overall well-being. Whether you're sipping on a vibrant green smoothie or indulging in a refreshing fruit juice, each sip is an investment in your health, offering a delicious way to fortify Provides your body with necessary vitamins, minerals, and antioxidants.

As you continue on your journey, I encourage you to experiment with the recipes and tailor them to your preferences and nutritional needs. Remember, every glass you raise to your lips is a toast to your health and vitality.

Once again, thank you for your time, your dedication, and your commitment to prioritizing your health. Here's to strong bones, radiant health, and a future filled with vitality.

With gratitude,

[LEONA BUTLER]

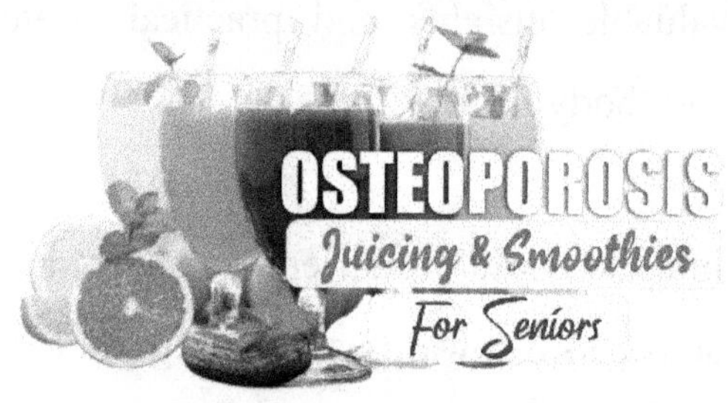

MY WEEKLY MEAL PLANNER

Date

	Breakfast	Lunch	Dinner
MON			
TUE			
WED			
THU			
FRI			
SAT			
SUN			

SHOPPING LIST:

To Do List

NOTES
AND TIPS

MY WEEKLY MEAL PLANNER

Date

	Breakfast	Lunch	Dinner
Mon			
Tue			
Wed			
Thu			
Fri			
Sat			
Sun			

SHOPPING LIST:

To Do List

Notes And Tips

MY WEEKLY MEAL PLANNER

Date

	Breakfast	Lunch	Dinner
Mon			
Tue			
Wed			
Thu			
Fri			
Sat			
Sun			

SHOPPING LIST:

To Do List

-
-
-
-

Notes
And Tips

MY WEEKLY MEAL PLANNER

Date

	Breakfast	Lunch	Dinner
MON			
TUE			
WED			
THU			
FRI			
SAT			
SUN			

SHOPPING LIST:

To Do List

- ●
- ●
- ●
- ●

NOTES
AND TIPS

MY WEEKLY MEAL PLANNER

Date

	Breakfast	Lunch	Dinner
MON			
TUE			
WED			
THU			
FRI			
SAT			
SUN			

SHOPPING LIST:

-
-
-
-

To Do List

NOTES
AND TIPS

MY WEEKLY MEAL PLANNER

Date

	Breakfast	Lunch	Dinner
MON			
TUE			
WED			
THU			
FRI			
SAT			
SUN			

SHOPPING LIST:

TO DO LIST

NOTES
AND TIPS

MY WEEKLY MEAL PLANNER

Date

	Breakfast	Lunch	Dinner
MON			
TUE			
WED			
THU			
FRI			
SAT			
SUN			

SHOPPING LIST:

To Do List

NOTES
AND TIPS

MY WEEKLY MEAL PLANNER

Date

	Breakfast	Lunch	Dinner
MON			
TUE			
WED			
THU			
FRI			
SAT			
SUN			

SHOPPING LIST:

To Do List

NOTES
AND TIPS

MY WEEKLY MEAL PLANNER

Date

	Breakfast	Lunch	Dinner
MON			
TUE			
WED			
THU			
FRI			
SAT			
SUN			

SHOPPING LIST:

-
-
-
-

TO DO LIST

NOTES
AND TIPS

MY WEEKLY MEAL PLANNER

Date

	Breakfast	Lunch	Dinner
Mon			
Tue			
Wed			
Thu			
Fri			
Sat			
Sun			

SHOPPING LIST:

To Do List

- ·
- ·
- ·
- ·

Notes
And Tips

MY WEEKLY MEAL PLANNER

Date

	Breakfast	Lunch	Dinner
MON			
TUE			
WED			
THU			
FRI			
SAT			
SUN			

SHOPPING LIST:

-
-
-
-

TO DO LIST

NOTES
AND TIPS

MY WEEKLY MEAL PLANNER

Date

	Breakfast	Lunch	Dinner
MON			
TUE			
WED			
THU			
FRI			
SAT			
SUN			

SHOPPING LIST:

TO DO LIST

NOTES
AND TIPS

MY WEEKLY MEAL PLANNER

Date

	Breakfast	Lunch	Dinner
MON			
TUE			
WED			
THU			
FRI			
SAT			
SUN			

SHOPPING LIST:

To Do List

-
-
-
-

NOTES
AND TIPS

MY WEEKLY MEAL PLANNER

Date

	Breakfast	Lunch	Dinner
MON			
TUE			
WED			
THU			
FRI			
SAT			
SUN			

SHOPPING LIST:

- ....
- ....
- ....
- ....

TO DO LIST

....
....
....
....

NOTES
AND TIPS